Bernhard Johannes Schmidt

PLAINTEXT
compact

The ASPERGER Syndrome

for Parents

Bernhard J. Schmidt

PLAINTEXT compact
The ASPERGER Syndrome
for Parents

© 2019 Bernhard J. Schmidt,
Oberwarmensteinach, Gemany
All Rights reserved.

ISBN: 978-3750417861

translated from
KLARTEXT kompakt
Das ASPERGER Syndrom – für Eltern
© 2015 Bernhard J. Schmidt
ISBN: 978 373 9216034

Production and Publishing:
BoD – Books on Demand, Norderstedt, Germany
Bibliographic information of the German National Library:
The German National Library lists this publication
in the German National Bibliography; detailed bibliographic
Data are available online at http://dnb.dnb.de.

Table of content

I. To get you started 2

II. Foreword..6

III. Odyssey..8

IV. The socio-cultural environment 10

V. The autistic communication 12

VI. Autists communicate different! 15

VII. With and Without „Autopilot".....................17

VIII. Anxiety and Stress......................................19

IX. The „Task-Mode"..21

X. Hypersensitivity...25

XI. Autismus Spectrum.......................................27

XII. Aspie memories..29

XIII. Finale...54

XIV. Bibliography:...55

I. TO GET YOU STARTED

You as a parent of an Asperger child
have a high probability of suffering from stress, social
phobia, depression, anxiety disorders ...

because you

- – want the best for your child, but understand it
  (almost) not.

- – experienced rejection and exclusion by friends,
  environment and relatives ...

- – seek help and support as well as explanation for
  the nature of your child.

- – but mostly experience incompetence and
  disinterest by diagnostics, school authorities,
  schools ...

- – must endure long waits for doctors and
  authorities and the feeling of helplessness.

- are accused that your child is not autistic, but you have only educated it wrongly.

- have (unconscious) expectations of your child who can not fulfill it (!)

- live with worries and fears for the future of your child.

- suffer from the exclusion your child experiences on a daily basis.

Your child

- would like to communicate (with you) - just does it differently, in his own way.

- want to interact with you - just in a different (his own) way.

- needs social (!) contacts - like any other child - to his development.

- will develop - only on a very own way.

- needs you as a reliable (!) companion.

- needs a clear structure and communication to find his way around.

- has the same needs as other kids too.

- has to master the same hurdles and transitions as other children - but not as part of a group, but alone.

- experiences exclusion, marginalization, accusations just like you - just much more intense.

- Perceives the world around you as you - only much more intense.

- has many strengths to discover and to promote.

- needs much more energy than other children and is therefore quickly exhausted, the "battery" is quickly empty.

- When your child is at the end of his power, you will not be able to reach him - then he just needs rest or retreat.

- has two big enemies: fear and stress.

Feel your fear, your stress. Both have a negative effect on you and your child.

II. FOREWORD

Autistic communication is different!
If a neurologically typical person (NT person) wrote this book, it would certainly have at least five times the scope. Autists talk plainly, NT people express themselves rather rambling and out of focus.

Thus, this book is not only the representation of problems and opportunities in the education of an Asperger child, but is also also an example and expression of autistic communication.

The decision for this book came from the discussions with parents of Asperger children after my lectures as well as in the autism consultation.

Here again and again I came across the same problems, misunderstandings and questions.

So far, because of a false static, isolated and cognitive psychological view, there were (too) many but unhelpful and contradictory answers.

The new social as well as the developmental psychological viewpoint makes many causes of the problems of and dealing with autistic people understandable, the many questions parents ask, why their Asperger children behave either way, can be conclusively answered.

To understand one's child is one of the central desires and goals of parents - and understanding is also the best help. Contributing to this is the goal of this book.

The fact that not all points and questions can be explained with the topic "autism", certainly not in such a brief representation, is unavoidable and also not goal. More information about autism, the new view, etc. can be found on my homepage

www.autismusberatung.info

and in my books "Understanding Autism" as well as "Helping Autistics?" (see bibliographie at the end of the book).
There you will also find detailed descriptions of current scientific research, errors in previous autism research as well as extensive references and further literature.

III. ODYSSEY

In conversation with parents of AS children (AS = autism spectrum) unfortunately the descriptions of catastrophic diagnostic processes are repeated. Diagnoses are rejected, problems are downplayed, parents are described as incapable of education, long waiting times have to be bridged, long paths are taken for a diagnosis become. When the diagnosis of "Asperger Autism" finally comes after long trials and tribulations, the odyssey continues. Although the diagnosis often leads to a relief in the parents, because they have a name for the many problems and now also a claim for support. However, the questions "What is autism" and "What can we do?" are not answered at all, wrongly or superficially. Parents suddenly need to know and accept that their child actually has a diagnosis that sees society as a disability. In principle, parents do not expect that they will have a child with "disability". They need to say goodbye to the idea of a child with a "normal" CV, go through a period of mourning: that does not mean that one is sad or disappointed with their child, but that a whole new phase of life starts with completely unexpected and unknown tasks. And that one must say goodbye to his previous ideas and habits.

8

Support must be won by parents - at the youth welfare office, kindergarten, school, teachers, kindergarten teachers, school assistants ... who, in most cases, do not even know what autism is.

Often parents of AS children do not encounter support but a lot of incompetence, disinterest and rejection. This rejection is often experienced in their own family environment, with friends and acquaintances. Not only the AS child with its non-social behaviors is rejected, but also his parents. Thus, parents of AS children (ie you!) have a greatly increased risk, e.g. to suffer from social phobia, depression, anxiety disorders, stress-related problems.

The same rejections are experienced by AS children and have the same risk with respect to the above-mentioned diseases and health problems. But moreover, as children who are not yet settled, they have yet to develop - much more so than their parents.

What you experience in terms of incompre-hension, accusations, rejection, etc. - your AS child also suffers every day! Only much more intense.

IV. THE SOCIO-CULTURAL ENVIRONMENT

The autism spectrum is referred to as "pervasive developmental disorder". It has been overlooked to this day that "development" is not static but dynamic. And second, in a socio-cultural environment.

Just as the process of diagnosis depends on the people and institutions you meet as parents, so does the development of the AS child depend on its environment! In a Tibetan (with prayer wheels) Buddhist monastery, an autistic person will not be noticed - and if positive then! Why?

Because there are few sensory stimuli in a monastery, little to no talk at all, much (actually the whole routine of the day) is ritualized and structured ... and the soothing turning of the prayer wheels is an accepted behavior.

Many strange behaviors of your child are a "substitute" for turning the prayer wheels!

But we do not live in Tibet, not in a monastery - but in a technological prosperity society. The recurring questions of parents of AS children are:

"How can my child develop as positively and

comprehensively as possible in this society?" And "What is contrary to a development of my child? What are the hurdles and obstacles? "

With a dynamic perspective before the respective socio-cultural background, one thing quickly becomes clear: Autism is NOT a developmental disorder, but through the interaction and communication (which is actually the same!) With the respective environment lead to a developmental disorder!

Not to move out of home until mid-forties, preferring to listen to Christmas carols all year round, not have had a boyfriend and girlfriend, and been in sustained therapy dependency, what e.g. Miss Dr. Preissmann, a german autism author and psychotherapist, describes from her life is NOT a necessary development! It's just one of many possible developments.

Everyone needs social (!) communication to develop and unfold their personality.
But depending on the environment, people who are perceived as "different" because they are not "socially compliant" and above all communicate differently, are marginalized and attacked. Not only the AS-child withdraws (mostly for good, comprehensible reasons!), but it is also often rejected and excluded from communication.

V. THE AUTISTIC COMMUNICATION

To understand what makes autistic communication
different, it is important to realize that communication is
multi-layered.
Part of our communication skills is innate (such as the
ability to speak, to learn a language). On the other hand,
another part must be learned, such as the language of my
environment. This learning is not so much about learning
the words and grammar as it is for the VHS course, but
about integrating them into a common cultural basis, the
"common ground". This common cultural basis is
therefore learned and is the basis of e.g. also for the
understanding of metaphors, proverbs etc.
Autists who find it difficult to understand metaphors and
proverbs have not (sufficiently) developed the "common
ground" of communication due to a lack of experience!
Who like Dr. med. Preissmann does not adequately
behave in a social situation and / or dress (sandales and
tracksuit for the wedding of the brother) lacks experience
in dealing with other people. These problems are
therefore not inherently autistic, but arise from
insufficient participation in communicative processes.
On the other hand, one must distinguish conscious and
unconscious communication. NT people always try to

uphold the image of the "conscious, rational and autonomous acting man" (CRAAM dogma), but social psychology shows different results.

NT people communicate to a large extent unconsciously, non-verbally, so not linguistically, but by facial expressions, gestures, modulation of the tuning melody, imitation, synchronization ...

Through this unconscious communication the affiliation to the group, the hierarchy in the group, sympathy and antipathy etc. are mediated.

Anyone who regards language in particular and communication in general by NT people only as a means of communication, overlooks an essential function: The distinction of in-group and out-groups. Whether you "belong" or not. Whether one speaks the same dialect, or that of the neighboring village a few kilometers away. Scientists estimate that about 60-70% of NT communication consists of gossip. Namely for the purpose of modern grooming, ie the strengthening of the sense of belonging to one's own group.

Much of the communication of neurologically typical people is therefore unconscious, serves the group definition and determination of the hierarchy, the orientation through and within the group. This communication is NOT "social" but group related! And this group communication consists not only of the content / messages sent, but also the expectations of the person, the nature and the extent of his messages.

So if one side "grooms" the other through conscious and unconscious communication, then of course this is also expected in return.

What is sent out as (unconscious) communication is also expected from the other person.

VI. AUTISTS COMMUNICATE DIFFERENT!

Autistic people lack all unconscious group communication, be it gossip, facial expressions, gestures, imitation ...

Autists communicate subject matter - almost 100% - they speak plain text. Therefore, they are usually quite silent even compared to NT people.
And autistic people expect exactly the same thing-oriented form of communication from their counterpart. (Unconscious) group communication they can not or only with great difficulty decrypt.

Talk to your AS child as concisely, clearly and objectively as possible.

A problem of our society is that we got used to an almost continuous "psycho-babbel". Statements like "You, that somehow makes me a bit affected. But it's good that we talked openly a bit about it." you will find unfortunately not only in various comedy programs. Your AS child can not and will not understand this "babbel"! (But as an AS adult after a sufficient participation in the socio-cultural environment its possible.)

The communication of autistic people is a bit harsh and unfriendly, because both the unconscious part of the communication through facial expressions, gestures and imitation as well as the "grooming" by gossip are missing.

The supposed "lack of empathy" that is often mistakenly attributed to autistics is simply the absence of unconscious group communication!

Autists even feel more intense with their fellow humans than NT people. If your child tells you something about his special interests, that's a sign of affection!

BE AWARE that the lack of unconscious (group) communication in your child does not mean repulse or rejection from you.

Since your AS child can not participate in subconscious group communication and does not understand it, in many cases it also needs clear and clear feedback in order to be able to orient oneself!

Do not expect that your AS-child will notice or sense whether it did something wrong or right, good or bad, you love it and like it - tell it clearly!

VII.   WITH AND WITHOUT „AUTOPILOT"

The unconscious group communication acts like an autopilot for NT people. Due to the unconscious orientation to the group, many decisions do not have to be made with great effort. This has Digby Tantam, an American doctor and autism researcher nicely formulated in his book (2009) „Can the world afford autistic spectrum disorder? Nonverbal communication, asperger syndrome and the interbrain.":

„... linked together by an endless chain to which we become attached when we are born and from which we only escape when we die. The chain may be a fetter, like the leg irons, but it also keeps us going in the same direction as anyone else, and at the same pace. People with ASD are not, I imagine, chained. They are free but they are also outside of the system. They can diverge from the norm, and many of them do, but the price that they pay is that they are not part of the solid mass of the group."

The (unconscious) orientation of the group also serves as both an "energy-saving mode" and the reduction of anxiety and stress.

17

Without unconscious group communication, autistics lack the "autopilot". This means a considerable amount of energy and time for orientation. Your AS-child does not just swim in the crowd, but has to create its own structure and decide on a direction.

Help your child through clear structures and clear boundaries, through a clear "yes" and a clear "no".

Structures and clear boundaries provide security and guidance. Again, our society has developed unhelpful ideas and behaviors. As early as 1973 Erik Erikson mocked in his book "Identity and Life Cycle - Three Essays." about this development with the formulation of the question "You, Mum, do I have to play today again what I want?"

Create within safe limits but also free spaces in which your AS child can build up and try out his own structures and orientations.

VIII. ANXIETY AND STRESS

The lack of unconscious group communication leads to anxiety and stress in your AS child in several ways. Yes, anxiety and stress are even the biggest problems for your AS child and can severely hamper his development.

The reduction of anxiety and stress is always the top priority.

But how do you get anxiety and stress?
On the one hand, people with their group behavior appear unpredictable and irrational to the AS child. That causes anxiety.
On the other hand, the AS child always has to re-orient himself with much effort of time and energy. With practice, this is getting easier - but in the beginning it is a rocky road.
At the same time, because of the lack of group communication, it is often rejected, marginalized or attacked by other people and groups.
Especially in adolescence, even if the AS-teenager tries to orientate himself on peers, his own inability to communicate with groups often becomes painfully clear to him, without, however, knowing why it does not work.

In some groups for AS-teenagers participation is worse, in others it is better. This essentially depends on whether the group is task-oriented and clearly structured or not.

The best way to participate is in groups that are task-oriented, structured, and have a clear hierarchy, such as the voluntary fire brigades, the Red Cross, ...

NT people compulsively and unconsciously follow an in-group / outgroup distinction. By this unconscious assignment of other people arise on the one hand (often unconsciously) prejudices.
These are missing from your AS child as well as the group assignment.
On the other hand, the words and deeds of the fellow human beings are evaluated by NT people depending on the group affiliation. Members of the own group are better rated and preferred. Members of outgroups, on the other hand, tend to be rejected, regardless of the accuracy, e.g. a statement or action.
By contrast, AS people are not interested in who says something, but what they say is of interest. The qualitative benefits that result from the lack of unconscious group communication Attwood and Gray reported in 1999 in their "Criteria for the Discovery of Aspie."

IX. THE „TASK-MODE"

Neurologically typical people have two possible states, the

- Task mode and the

- Relaxation mode (default mode).

The task mode is intended for the management of problems and tasks, the relaxation mode for the (unconscious) group communication, the "grooming". The relaxation mode is characterized by superficiality, orientation to the group, gossip, in-group / outgroup discrimination ...

In a prosperous society, NT people live mainly in the relaxation mode. And that even if problems actually have to be solved. The skyrocketing of the number of talk shows in crises shows this impressively.

On the other hand, AS humans only have the task mode, they can not switch to the relaxation mode.

So your AS child is in a continuous activity mode. It has real interest already in its early years.

On the nature, technology or his other special interest. In addition, the child knows (often already at the age of four

21

years) amazingly much.

The relaxation mode of NT people, however, is foreign to the AS child. The simple question is, "What's that for?" Due to the lack of unconscious group communication, the relaxation mode remains a mystery to the AS child. Be it in the school break, on excursions without content-related goal ...

However, everything connected with a task, a factual content, is just right. The excursion to a museum, the exploration of caves ...

An AS child, who is normally barely able to get out, will be able to overcome his or her own fears and inhibitions in order to obtain information or solve a problem.

The royal road to participation and activity, to reassure and satisfy your AS child is a task to be solved!

NT people in relaxation mode, however, show no interest but superficiality. The AS child, on the other hand, who really wants to get to the bottom of things, then seems difficult, slow, inattentive ...

The learning that results from solving problems, ie the learning of your AS child, is called "emulation learning". This requires several things:

- The presence of a real problem.

- The interest in solving this problem.

Anything that your AS child is interested in will he learn at lightning speed because he's always in the task mode. And he will always look for new tasks.

Recognize and promote the interests of your AS child. Also awaken new areas of interest!

NT people in default mode, on the other hand, learn mainly through imitation, that is imitating what, for example, a teacher is doing. A real interest or desire to solve problems is missing.

Schools and school systems that are not based on superficiality and imitation, but that foster the interest of the AS child (such as Montessori schools), and where there is also scope for individual problem-solving strategies, are best for your AS child.

Many AS children had to change schools several times and sometimes change school assistants in order to reach a satisfactory school situation. You should not shy away from the effort involved, because attending school for many years is the essential part of participating in groups and cultural environments. Here, among other things, the foundation stone is laid for either a further positive personal development or the development of a personality disorder.

Due to the lack of "relaxation mode", holidays and weekends are often problematic for AS children.

For NT people holidays are relaxing, for people with autism they often mean stress, because the regular daily routine and the structure are missing. On top of that, doing nothing for AS children can mean sheer stress.

X. HYPERSENSITIVITY

No, even though presented by the media and some autistic people, a combination of ADHD, hypersensitivity and narcissism is NOT autism!

"Autism" is the term for the previously described lack of unconscious group communication!

And with it comes however an increased sensory sensitivity, thus with the perceptions of seeing, hearing, smelling, feeling.

Among the problems that result from the lack of the "autopilot" are thus added to the problems of this hypersensitivity aggravating.

Things that you can not hear, see or smell can cause your AS child to become overloaded.

If possible, borrow some hearing aids, set them to maximum volume, and walk around with them.

Experiencing the associated stress, the inability to filter out voices from the total noise, etc., matches what your AS child perceives. Added to this is the increased perception of light, e.g. the flickering of a neon tube that you do not even notice. The perception of (unpleasant) smells ...

Through these intense perceptions, your AS child is easily under constant stress.

A withdrawal of your child or an overreaction often have their cause in excessive sensory stimuli.

If your AS child gets too much due to overstimulation, then the "Tilt" sign will appear as it did in the pinball machine. And without an appropriate regeneration phase, your AS child will not be ready and able to communicate or interact. So give your child a break or avoid overloading.

The sensory stimuli of the environment, whether at home or at school, etc., you should pay the utmost attention. What you normally filter out automatically, you can certainly be aware of, if you pay attention.

In addition, strong sensory stimuli (as well as touch!) can cause anxiety when they are perceived as threatening or overwhelming.

XI. AUTISMUS SPECTRUM

While one used to differentiate between Asperger syndrome, Kanner autism (infantile autism) and HFA (high-functioning autism), today one assumes an autism spectrum. Unfortunately, this is called "disorder". The underlying problem is that the autism researchers did not look beyond the area of "diagnosis" that presupposes suffering, and do not look beyond. However, the autism spectrum goes beyond limiting to diagnosed autistic individuals. Unfortunately, those who have gone their own way, found their place in society, do not appear neither in research nor in public perception.

The fate of your AS child is therefore not sealed as in people with permanent, irreversible damage. Your child can also become diagnosed in the sense that it is still autistic, but does not suffer from it. So an "Aspie" with the benefits of clear thinking, loyalty, honesty, reliability ... and no Asperger Autist with diagnosis. Your child can also find his place in society and live independently and happy.

This should be the goal of your efforts. You should not let the belief in a good future for your AS child deter you, even if obstacles and resistance sometimes seem insurmountable.

The goal of a contented life in which your child can unfold his abilities and personality - and not necessarily be adapted to socially desired behavior.

To reason and freedom as a goal, you can not force your AS-child, you can only open the door and show the way. In order not to make this appear as empty promises or false hopes, and as a counterpole to the many publications of autistics that confuse their social phobia, anxiety disorders, narcissism, etc. with autism, a brief account of my own past follows. The road was not always easy and was associated with several detours and lows. But it has led me to a state of balance and freedom that has enabled me in recent years to develop all my creative and intellectual abilities.

XII.   ASPIE MEMORIES

Sempre avanti
Memories of an Aspie

I was born in 1962 in Dortmund, Germany, where I spent my childhood and youth.

My father, also Aspie, was a lawyer and notary, incorruptible, not corruptible and always independent of the "opinion" of others.

At a time when "environmental protection" did not exist and Mercedes was considered a status symbol, he was already cycling or walking.

Even after long holidays, while stopping and waiting for the night train in Munich, we went (and we all looked like the robbers) anyway in the finest and best restaurants. The holidays we spent over many years and decades always in the same pension in Bad Reichenhall, Bavaria. Even then I realized that whenever we went to the mountains I felt physically better.

Olfactory horror

The elementary school passed by in a rather unspectacular way ... except for physical education.

As an aspie, sport is not exactly a feast by itself, but far worse was a girl with surname Sp ..., who always sat in the team either behind or in front of me. She wore always, no matter winter or summer, woolen tights ... and always smelled unwashed, sweet as if putrefaction. I still have the smell in my nose today, and remind me too well of the feeling of disgust and the horror of physical education.

In order to promote me, my parents had also registered me in a sports club, whose construction is no longer today and had already been demolished. The dressing room was "Sp ... square", the sports hall no better.

No, sport was not really my thing, but at least later that should change at times.

Social competence or "Task-Positive-Network"

The high school went - largely unnoticed by me - over. Without wanting to do so, I have sometimes driven my brothers and parents to the brink of madness, because my favorite activity was "lying on the bed, staring blanket and doing nothing".

At some point my parents gave me the book "The Adventures of the Strong Wanja" by Ottfried Preußler. But I'm not sure if it was more about encouraging me or them.

When I was not lying on my bed and staring at the blanket, I was very active in Catholic youth work. First group leader, then parish youth leader, with 17 then led the first of three tent camps. Camping meant to camp with about 50 children and teenagers for 14 days. A social as well as a logistical and organizational challenge. But there was not a single critical situation in the three camps!

The authorities, offices and applications all knew me at the time, because I applied for each grant, I knew each form by heart, whether 50 cents per person per day for "church elements in youth work" or subsidies for the purchase of new tents ...

Tasks and challenges, that were the keys to my well-being even then. And that was always connected to the ability to deal with people, indeed many people. Insignificance or small-talk I can not stand. But actively leading a group, working together to solve tasks - that's a celebration.

Loss of sheltered childhood and youth

There was nothing for me to do but refuse military service. At that time there was still the "examination of conscience", which of course I did not pass. Then the examination in front of the "committee of conscience", of

31

course I failed. And so it came to the action before the Administrative Court "Bernhard Schmidt against the Federal Republic of Germany" ... "It issued the following sentence: The action is granted." Reads now maybe rather funny. but for me it was a very serious break. I was aware that my entire future will depend on the verdict. The feeling of powerlessness tore me vehemently out of my sheltered childhood and youth.

Sempre Avanti - or the aspie imperative

Sempre avanti - that was always my father's invitation to me ... always moving forward! And so came from him the proposal to make my civil service in Bad Reichenhall. A good chance to get away from home.

With work and a roof over my head, a limited time ... and Bad Reichenhall, which I already knew through our many holidays.

So on to Reichenhall, the Red Cross ... and off in the disabled service.

It was the most educational and beautiful time of my life. The handling of people with disabilities has changed me a lot. Who is complaining of a cold over someone who is sitting in a wheelchair from birth but is in a good mood. The values have shifted very much since then with me. But driving service was called driving about 200km a day. So it was normal that I came over, sometimes serious, car accidents again and again. But from first aid I had no idea.

After a short conversation with the district manager, he then sent me to the 6-week rescue service training.

No sooner was I back from training in Reichenhall, I came in Salzburg to an accident in which a boy had been hit. The CPR of the boy on the street has shown me clearly that the theory of rescue service training is not enough.

So I often volunteered 24 hours a day - daytime disabled service, at night volunteer rescue service. The rescue service led to a tough encounter with the topic of death and at the same time to a cross-sectional study by the population. You get into many apartments, the poor as well as the rich. You get into the most absurd situations and learn about suicides that are never in the newspaper.

They are funny animals, people

This was clearly shown to me in the Festspielhaus in Salzburg. A customer of the handicapped driver service with severe visual impairment was driven by me more frequently to operas and concerts and also accompanied. An accumulation of many people is now nothing that an aspie wants. But these experiences surpassed everything.

My idea that it would be about culture and therefore cultivated people and therefore could not be so bad, was quickly refuted. A jostling, pushing ... worse than on the fairground. Bringing a visually impaired woman through unscathed was always a Herculean task. And that, even though everyone had a reserved place. Similar experiences of irrational and asocial behavior of NT's, however, I have then again and again make "allowed".

"no-group" instead of "no sports"

After the civil service, the question was: what to do? A vocational training was out of the question, unfortunately. So study, but what? My wish would have been actually medicine (high school diploma too bad) or philosophy (breadless art). So it became "physical engineering" at the University of Applied Sciences Lübeck.
The study did not really interest me, and so I became a quick sports referent in the ASTA (General Students Committee) than I could look. Was the previous ASTA from the classic "we are important here and you have nothing to say" variety, the new team was much more open-minded. That's how I lived out my "no-group" openness. In a few weeks, we not only had a huge range of sports activities, but even a philosophical seminar ... at a purely technical college.

I did not do much for that. If someone came and wanted a sports offer, the communication was actually a) always friendly and open and b) actually always the same:
Do you have an exercise / course leader? - Yes.
Do you have a hall? - no.
Ok, with this city employee you get a hall, if it does not work, come back and I'll help you! - OK!
Shortly afterwards, I was elected ASTA Chairman - Powerplay at its best.
I had a great team at my side and we did things that were considered "impossible". Against the already planned cuts in the education sector, we managed a merger of administration, professors and students. Everyone was pulling together and there were strikes against the budget cuts. But do not just stay home and do nothing, but with "alternative strike weeks". We asked the professors what they always wanted to teach, but never happens in the curriculum. These were the best lectures I was able to experience in my life!

Meaning crisis, the shortest dropout of all time, and the courage to reverse

At some point I had to admit that I can not remain the chairman of the ASTA for the rest of my life and that my studies had already stopped. In addition, the experiences from the civil service worked hard, I asked myself intensively the question of the meaning of life.

Why not try the "alternative" life?

I had an address from an association in Austria that managed abandoned mountain farms alternatively.

So I quit my apartment, sold or gave away all the belongings, and gave myself up to the Austrian mountains.

But what awaited me there, I really had not expected. Narrow-mindedness, ignorance ... actually I wanted to go there on the first day. Everything was super important. Only they, the elect, were capable.

With a flock of sheep a part of the group moved in the summer through Austria and sold homemade teas. Original soundtrack of a resident "But we do not drink it ourselves - we do not know what's in there."

They also had a few cows and I was asked if I would come to the stable with them. There they left me like wrong money. But when I left, it was not right either.

But the worst thing for me, as an Aspie, who supposedly can not read feelings of faces and has no empathy, was the look in the eyes of a few residents who were far too clear to read that they were not happy there, but probably did not have the courage to go away.

It was different with me. On the second day, when nothing was better but actually everything got worse, I drove away. Quite in the knowledge of what I am allowed to listen to ("we knew that soon ...") and how one or the other will make fun of me.

It's hard to go your own way without sometimes leaving

Going away is good ... but where to go?
No apartment, no destination, no plan ... absolute zero, at the age of 25, without vocational training, without perspective ... as an aspie (which I did not know then)
First of all, I annoyed my longtime friend Arne for three weeks, who was living in a tiny loft apartment.

Freedom is just another word for nothing left to lose (Janis Joplin)

So what to do with maximum freedom? The thing I always wanted to do was to study philosophy. So back to Dortmund, an apartment and used furniture from friends and acquaintances found themselves faster than it had taken to get rid of the old furniture. Ruhr-University-Bochum, philosophy as a major subject and psychology and neurophysiology as minor subjects, that's what I thought, and so it was in the study guide as a possibility. But much is allowed or not prohibited just because nobody claims it. And so here too. It took me 6 months to get to grips with the student secretariat until it gave in and let me study my dream combination.

Psycho-lie and ambivalence

Rarely have I met another group as intolerant as the psychology students. I was treated frequently like air or with open refusal ...
I was not comfortable with them.
A fellow student also lived in Dortmund and we drove together several times to the university. On the way I was able to talk to her super, she was a pediatric nurse, I used to be in the rescue service ... similar attitudes, values ...
But once we were in the seminar, I was air. As if we had never met before.
And then such people become psychologists and therapists ...

The Rat King ...

In order to finance my studies, I had a position as a research assistant in a work unit of biopsychology. There I supervised the EDP and performed learning and labyrinth experiments with rats. A rat had inflammation on its head and had to be treated with ointment. So my colleague tried to stroke the wound ointment on the rat with a cotton swab. But no chance. the rat squirmed so that the ointment landed everywhere but not on the wound.

Trying makes sense, so I tried my luck. And ... as soon as I grabbed the rat (you can grasp it at the tail root), the rat became silent, stretched out all fours and I could calmly stroke the ointment on her head.

From then on I was considered the rat king, which did not make it easier for me to deal with my colleagues. Conversely, I would have preferred it.

... Dog Whisperer

Already in the civilian service, my special skills in dealing with animals became clear to me. In dealing with animals, there are these communication problems as with people just not. On the contrary, animals seem to understand and like the clear signals of an aspie.

While the full-time employee for "eating on wheels" was on vacation, I not only had the representation but also a new customer. Far out in the country, a stand-alone farmhouse with a huge, fenced yard around it. And a big sign "Warning to the dog". But there was no bell and cell phones did not exist then ... so what to do?

I had already seen the lurking dog, but what the hell, he

can not bite me more than that ;-)

So in the garden and the front door. The dog was lurking at a distance, but I had an incredulous and surprised-looking landlady in front of me. "So far no one has managed to leave the dog unmolested in the garden! How did you do that????"

The same asked me again the full-time official, when he was back from vacation.

… and auto mechanic

The second financial pillar during the study was repairing cars. And yes, I was really good. He enjoyed the recognition of fellow mechanics and was well known to the aftermarket dealers. I bought used cars without TÜV cheap. I then prepared these and sold them to friends and acquaintances. The inert gas welder and the angle grinder were my best friends ;-)

I started with 18 when I got my first own car. So I first repaired my own car, then made inspections for friends ... Then there was a 1963 folding roof beetle, Karman Ghia, Mercedes / 8, Hanomag Markant, Tempo Matador, Opel Rekord C, VW 1600 and 412LE, Mercedes LA710 ... in total over 30 own cars and many more from friends.

Study - End without degree

The study was coming to an end, all the notes in the bag, many good to very good grades. For example, Neurophysiology 45 minutes oral exam: very good.
It was missing "only" the master's thesis.
But suddenly there was no light that shone. The work unit where I had my job was closed. I could not find a supervisor of my MA thesis.
Well, with the topic "ethical problems with brain transplants" I was years ahead of my time. The one professors reacted to my request rather indignant, the other openly admitted that they had no idea about the subject area.
The medical professor had already considered giving me a PhD position, but then he did not dare. A philosopher - where so many medical students hoped for such a position! So what do you do?

Therapy

No, not for me. But for children and adolescents with food addiction (obesity). I was once again in Reichenhall, visiting friends (yes, you can also have them as an aspie). These worked in a rehab center for addicted children and were looking for an educator.

After 10 days of vacation, I came home with a signed contract of employment and a lease. It can go so fast. It followed the most intense 6 months of my life. Acceptance interviews, discussions with parents, individual therapy, group therapy, conflicts within the team, with the direction, abysses of human existence.

Rat catcher

The children and adolescents were a bit disturbed in the beginning, so I did not live up to the image of the soft, long-haired do-gooder. But I had learned that sometimes it takes time for the ice to break when dealing with me. After that, I had the best relationship and the most authority in the house among the children and adolescents. But I was not at all entitled to it! And I dork did not consider that.

The kids had stolen the chef's keychain and this was a big problem. What to do? Swap all locks? All punish? House meeting! And Schmidt explains the alternatives to the children: The keys return anonymously or the locks are exchanged. The bunch of keys came back the same evening, problem solved.

But like the Pied Piper of Hamelin, people are not so happy and kind when the problem is solved. They are more offended that they did not make it themselves.

Zero point number three

After the existential shock in the conscientious objection and the failed alternative life on the farm, I once again stood in front of nothing. Because of growing conflicts in the team, whose solution none of me wanted to tackle, and my unwillingness to tell the children to solve their problems and to get rid of the sick and fatiguing structures without doing it myself as a team, I have then terminated.

I had my apartment only half a year, no more work, no vocational training ... at 32 years again with nothing in front of nothing. Freedom is just another word ...

And it goes even deeper

On the occasion of my termination, there was still a supervision. And all the other 10 people and also the supervisor (totally out of her role and offending her responsibility) burst into tears and called me the evil made flesh.

Fortunately, I was already more than used to rejection by others and groups. Otherwise I would have taken a rope and looked for a nice tree.

The "turn around"

At the time nobody would have given a chanterelle to my future. Most saw me end up under a bridge ...
But after six weeks of unemployment, on a Saturday afternoon, it came to me, probably out of boredom, to simply fax to a few copier dealers with the idea to open a copy shop. It was just such an idea, a pastime and I did not expect anything. But then everything went very fast, I could not get out of the number and on July 15, 1994, I opened my business "Copy & Computer Schmidt". With that, I found my niche, in which, as an "integrated outsider", I happily and contentedly lived my life for 22 years. The nicest comment of a bavarian customer was: "The Schmidt is indeed a Preiß' [Prussian] ... but a very nice." ;-)

No, it's not over yet ...

There is the aspie imperative "Get the butt up and see what there is to discover in the world!"

Freedom of expression and democracy

There was only one newspaper in Bad Reichenhall and no freedom of expression. The coverage at that time was one-sided, uncritical and censored. Critical letters were not printed ...

Many had their heads above alternatives, but all came to the conclusion "that's not possible".

But on the way to an FDP party congress (yes, I was then district chairman) broke my collar. Again a very bad, one-page article in the newspaper.

On the same day, a fellow campaigner and I started to write the first issue of "POLIS", the next day we finished and printed them. It was a DIN A4 sheet, folded on DIN A5, ridiculous ... have probably thought the Reichenhaller who have even taken note of it.

Ultimately, it has then become over 60 issues with some editions of 7,000 copies.

Communication?

No, Aspies can not * lol

An intern asked if I would take him. He had to prove 6 months internship for his computer science studies. Sure, we'll do it.

But how to deal with the intern? How to challenge him? "Let's have a chat"

From this idea came thousands of hours of programming (not from me, but from the first trainee, then a colleague and today a doctor of computer science) the Ruperti-

Chat. A regional chat with sometimes up to 8,000 page views - during the day!
We quickly put the support, administration and design of the chat in the hands of the young people. These have given themselves under appropriate admin rights, organized themselves, the chat and the Chatter cared for ... have logged off, if they had no time or desire more. 98% of that worked well and we only had to deal with the chat technically. If everyone talks badly about the youth - I believe in them ever since. They are proven to be able to take responsibility and organize themselves.
Then Facebook came and unfortunately blew us the light in no time.

Confession

It was during a conversation with two acquaintances in a cafe. I was 42 years old and said "I am autistic".
Somehow you always know that you are different. That things do not work the way they should. That you always have difficulties in mutual understanding. It's not that only the Aspies do not understand the "world", but the "world" does not understand the Aspies either.
Gudrun sent me an e-mail saying she did some research on autism and she found something that would suit me pretty well: Asperger syndrome.

That was a wave of realization for me. Why things were the way they were.

Big party

What drives you, who whispers to you?
In the fall of 2005, friends and I planned to organize a "Festival of Clubs" in Reichenhall. Not as commercial as the city festival, where everyone just wants to sell sausages and beer. No, a real family party on which the clubs present themselves with their offers.
None of us knew that on 2 January 2006, the ice rink would collapse and claim 15 deaths.
And once again I heard "this is not possible, no one comes to you, you have made too many enemies with the POLIS ... are a Preiß [prussian]"
Nevertheless, we have simply invited all clubs to a preparatory meeting. And I will never forget the evening. We sat in the big hall and did not know how many clubs will come, if any will come, if the whole thing will succeed.
When the meeting began, the hall was full. At the "Festival of Clubs", 43 clubs presented themselves in the summer of 2006 and celebrated the day together.
Together they organized the tasting of the visitors and shared the profit. Everything is organized and carried out

47

by an aspie who allegedly has such great difficulties with social communication ... that's the way it can be.
But success awakens envious people, arouses fears, someone could become too powerful.
So unfortunately it was the only "Festival of Clubs" in Reichenhall.

Sideline Host or Gastronomic Harakiri?

Why not rent a restaurant? Always complaining in the POLIS that nobody changes anything, that's not enough ... I thought.
So in November 2007 I leased Berggasthof Schroffen.
The Reichenhall restaurateurs certainly laughed half dead and gave me no 3 months. A newcomer, without any idea of the gastronomy. And to an object on which previously had some experienced hosts bloody noses.
Then the spinner starts even in winter, works with regional producers and cooks seasonally.
Today is normal ... back then that was almost too far ahead of time.

Systemizing - empathizing theory - REFUTED

Yes, this is what Simon Baron-Cohen calls his "theory", which claims that one thing or another is good. Or both only mediocre. Aspies are the "systemizer" with the "lack of empathy"

Wrong, Prof. Baron-Cohen!

To successfully run a problematic restaurant, you need both.

Organization of personnel and goods use, control of energy consumption, advertising and logistics at the highest level.

But also the sure feeling for the guest, his wishes and needs. The ability to respond to the guest.

We specialize in events (birthdays, weddings ...) with 60 - 120 guests, successful! Because I was always very aware of what my guests want and what responsibility I carry.

Unfortunately I was not renewed the lease and after two years the fun was over. The Schroffen stood empty for many years. Irrational decision in its purest form!

That's not possible!

Many have thought I was just a joker or gossip when I talked about the conditions in 2013.

1,000 nights a month in a small guesthouse in Inzell.

Mediated by a big travel agency. 14,50 EUR net per day per person for ALL: staff, energy, contributions, taxes, laundry, ...

And of course breakfast, coffee and cake, in the evening

3 course menu and from 6pm to 9pm wine and beer included.

Well, possibly with cheapest products, lowest quality, low-paid employees.

No, but with meat and sausage from a local butcher, fruits and vegetables from the local greengrocer, wine from the winery and beer from a local brewery. And with an average age of the staff of 57 years, all employed by social security.

But, just as an aspie and "systemizer" you can do it!

It was an exhausting but exciting experience.

In 6 months 6,000 overnight stays, 850 guests. From all over Germany. Couples, families, pensioners ... many interesting discussions, many insights.

But if I applied anywhere in the restaurant business - nobody would take me.

Good thing I have my own business and I do not have to apply.

Summary

The fact that today I am where I am, satisfied, balanced and physically as well as mentally healthy, has several causes.

On the one hand, my parents, who always supported me in what I wanted (even if they disagreed) and did not force me to do what they wanted.

In addition the good, longtime friends. Friends who understood me and were there for me, even if it was not always easy with me and still is.

Moving to an aspie-friendly environment. Here in Bad Reichenhall everything is manageable, quickly familiar. The clocks are slower and suits are worn only by bankers and insurance agents. It is calm, cool and shady - even in summer. You are fast and without any effort or stress in the forest, so in the cool shade with these fantastic smells.

Then the founding of my business 20 years ago, "my shop is my castle", which brought me independence. The possibility to organize things as they are good for me. And today, after more than 20 years, I still like to go to my shop every day.

And of course, my courage and my energy to take advantage of every opportunity that came my way to make new experiences. And the necessary portion of luck.

All of this took place or started when I did not know or had acknowledged that I was an aspie.

Curiosities

Although I have no IT, commercial or other training, I have been doing business successfully for 20 years (survival is success!) And have been able to train an employee as a "businessman for office communication". Without educator training, I worked as an educator and accompanied a good friend through her educator training. The accompaniment consisted in the preparation of her lectures, for which she always got at least one "very good".

Without being a restaurant or hotel professional I have managed the most difficult operations.

Without training as an editor, I have published a city magazine.

And without these certificates and training, my abilities will never be recognized in this society. Society is not based on what someone can do, but what certificates he has.

Lookouts

Gastronomy is simply my (late discovered) passion. And to continue with solving problems related to social engagement.

My big plan is a housing project for people in old-age poverty. The inn in Inzell should actually already become, which unfortunately did not work because of differences with the owners. But that does not stop me.

Sometimes things take time to mature, just like a good red wine.

Current status at the time of translation

In the meantime, I've given up my "Copy & Computer Schmidt" business in order to implement the "Solidar Hotel" project described in the book "Autistic and Society. An Angry Change of Perspective. Volume 1: Understanding Autism".

In the first two years of operation, we had over 300 families with more than 500 children, 50 of them autistic, as guests.

And it has been shown that my autism theory was and is right. The children showed some amazing developments by reducing anxiety and stress among them and their parents. These developmental advances have also come about through the possibility of social interaction with other children and adults. Social interaction is learned through social interaction!

Unfortunately I had to withdraw from the project in 2019 out of consideration for my health.

The experiences I've written down in the books "Autism and Dog", "Is my child Autistic? Encouraging answers to a scary question" and "Autism - flight or fight, new perspectives on challenging behavior".

XIII.   FINALE

Be your AS child

- **a "safe haven"**

- **a clear and reliable orientation**

- **a conversation partner in "Task Mode"**

Reduce stress and anxiety in both yourself and your AS child.

Encourage your AS-child to participate in groups, in society and in cultural events, even if it often fails.

Seek help and support in a support group or start one yourself. For the parents of AS children, social interaction, exchange of experiences and successes is an important basis for satisfaction and mental health. Do not lose your courage and commitment.

XIV.   BIBLIOGRAPHY:

Schmidt, Bernhard J. (2015/1): Autistic and Society. An angry Change of Perspective. Vol. I: **Understanding Autism**. Norderstedt: Books on Demand.

Schmidt, Bernhard J. (2015/2): Autistic and Society. An angry Change of Perspective. Vol. II: **Support for Autistic**? Norderstedt: Books on Demand.

Schmidt, Bernhard J. (2016): Plaintext compact. **The Asperger Syndrome – Between Bullying and Inclusion**. Norderstedt: Books on Demand.

Schmidt, Bernhard J.; Ganz, Andreas (2016): Plaintext compact: **The Asperger Syndrome - not only for Psychotherapists.** Norderstedt: Books on Demand.

Schmidt, Bernhard J.; Döhler, Christiane and Deniz (2018): **Autism – Sexuality – Relationships.** Norderstedt: Books on Demand.

Schmidt, Bernhard J. (2019): **Autism and the Refrigerator Mother Myth. A Rehabilitation of Bruno Bettelheim.** Norderstedt: Books on Demand.

Schmidt, Bernhard J. (2019): Plaintext compact. **The Asperger Syndrome – for Teachers.** Norderstedt: Books on Demand.

Schmidt, Bernhard J. (2019): Plaintext compact. **The Asperger Syndrome – for School Assistants.** Norderstedt: Books on Demand.

Schmidt, Bernhard J. (2019): Plaintext compact. **The Asperger Syndrome – for Physicians.** Norderstedt: Books on Demand.

Schmidt, Bernhard J. (2019): **Autism – Fight or Flight. New Perspectives on Challenging Behaviors.** Norderstedt: Books on Demand.